T0292262

# Manual of

# ANTERIOR SEGMENT SURGERY

# Manual of

# ANTERIOR SEGMENT SURGERY

**S. Gregory Smith, MD**
*Wilmington, Delaware*
*Former Attending Surgeon*
*Wills Eye Hospital*
*Philadelphia, Pennsylvania*

**Ryan G. Smith, MD**
*Los Altos, California*

**Richard L. Lindstrom, MD**
*Founder and Attending Surgeon, Minnesota Eye Consultants*
*Adjunct Professor Emeritus, Department of Ophthalmology*
*University of Minnesota*
*Minneapolis, Minnesota*
*Visiting Professor, Gavin Herbert Eye Institute*
*University of California, Irvine*
*Irvine, California*
*Global Medical Editor, Ocular Surgery News*

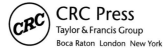

**CRC Press**
Taylor & Francis Group
Boca Raton  London  New York

CRC Press is an imprint of the
Taylor & Francis Group, an **informa** business

First published 2019 by SLACK Incorporated

Published 2024 by CRC Press
2385 NW Executive Center Drive, Suite 320, Boca Raton FL 33431

and by CRC Press
4 Park Square, Milton Park, Abingdon, Oxon, OX14 4RN

*CRC Press is an imprint of Taylor & Francis Group, LLC*

© 2019 Taylor & Francis Group, LLC

*Dr. S. Gregory Smith*, *Dr. Ryan G. Smith*, and *Dr. Richard L. Lindstrom* have no financial or proprietary interest in the materials presented herein.

Cover Artist: Lori Shields

Library of Congress Cataloging-in-Publication Data
Names: Smith, S. Gregory, author. | Smith, Ryan G., author. | Lindstrom,
   Richard L., author.
Title: Manual of anterior segment surgery / S. Gregory Smith, Ryan G. Smith,
   Richard L. Lindstrom.
Description: Thorofare : SLACK Incorporated, 2018. | Includes index.
Identifiers: LCCN 2018030110 (print) | ISBN 9781630916206 (pbk. : alk. paper)
Subjects: | MESH: Anterior Eye Segment--surgery | Microsurgery--methods |
   Ophthalmologic Surgical Procedures--methods
Classification: LCC RD33.6 (print) | NLM WW 210 | DDC
   617.05--dc23
LC record available at https://lccn.loc.gov/2018030110


ISBN: 9781630916206 (pbk)
ISBN: 9781003524984 (ebk)

DOI: 10.1201/9781003524984

# DEDICATION

This book is dedicated to our teachers, our students, and our colleagues. The virtuous covenant of one generation of physicians teaching the next to advance our field remains as critical as ever. We also want to thank our wives and family who have shared our journey in ophthalmology and provided unconditional love and support.

# Contents

# ABOUT THE AUTHORS

*S. Gregory Smith, MD* trained at the University of Minnesota in Minneapolis under Dr. Lindstrom from 1979 to 1983, including a fellowship in cornea and anterior segment surgery. He taught surgery and rose to the rank of Attending Surgeon at Wills Eye Hospital in Philadelphia, PA, where he practiced for over 20 years. Dr. Smith has had numerous publications in peer-reviewed journals, authored a previous textbook, *Complications of Intraocular Lenses and Their Management*, and has over 30 patents. He is currently in private practice in Wilmington, DE.

*Ryan G. Smith, MD* is completing his residency in ophthalmology at Stanford University in California. An avid photographer, this is his first venture in medical photography.

*Richard L. Lindstrom, MD* completed undergraduate, medical school, and residency training at the University of Minnesota and affiliated hospitals in 1977. He then pursued 2 years of fellowship training in cornea, ophthalmic microsurgery, and glaucoma in Minneapolis, MN, Dallas, TX, and Salt Lake City, UT. He is Founder and Attending Surgeon at Minnesota Eye Consultants, Clinical Professor Emeritus of Ophthalmology at the University of Minnesota, a University of Minnesota Foundation Trustee, Visiting Professor at the University of California, Irvine Gavin Herbert Eye Institute, and Global Chief Medical Editor of *Ocular Surgery News*.

Dr. Lindstrom is a board-certified ophthalmologist and internationally recognized leader in cornea, cataract, refractive, glaucoma, and laser surgery. He has been at the forefront of ophthalmology's evolutionary changes throughout his career as a recognized researcher, teacher, inventor, writer, lecturer, and highly acclaimed physician and surgeon. A frequent lecturer throughout the world, he has presented over 40 named lectures and keynote speeches. He has been awarded over 40 patents in ophthalmology and has developed a number of corneal preservation solutions, intraocular lenses, and instruments that are used in clinical practices globally. He has co-edited 7 books and published over 350 peer-reviewed journal articles and 60 book chapters. His professional affiliations are extensive.

# PREFACE

During our decades of teaching residents and fellows the nuances of ophthalmic microsurgery, we learned that appropriate hand positions are a foundational skill. Adapting and utilizing a small number of core hand positions allows the ophthalmic surgeon to more rapidly learn new maneuvers and perform them with reduced stress and a shorter learning curve. This small manual is our attempt to share these learnings and be there in the operating room with each of you as we all strive together to enhance our surgical skills.

# FOREWORD

With this text, *Manual of Anterior Segment Surgery*, the authors have decided to address a greatly overlooked aspect of this surgery: the set up, correct positioning, and ergonomics for the surgeon. With this text, the authors instruct us on the proper position of the hands, feet, and body during surgery. When learning surgical techniques, we are all taught to focus on what is transpiring in the eye itself, but this text will be instructing us on what is happening outside the eye. The authors take us step by step through the cataract procedure and point out the correct and most efficient way to position ourselves.

Drs. Gregory Smith and Richard Lindstrom are internationally known surgeons and authors. They both have taught us a great deal in their storied careers. They are respected teachers and innovators in cataract, corneal, and refractive surgery. Dr. Gregory Smith has a unique way of looking at problems and issues that many of us overlook and take for granted. The final author, Dr. Ryan Smith, is early in his career, but his perspective is a great asset to his co-authors.

This is a text that is current, concise, yet comprehensive. It will be invaluable to the beginning surgeon but also a great resource for experienced surgeons. I am confident this text will make us all better and more efficient surgeons. It will improve surgical care to the benefit of our patients.

Drs. Smith, Lindstrom, and Smith: thank you for addressing this important topic and sharing your wisdom and knowledge.

*Edward J. Holland, MD*
Director, Cornea Services
Cincinnati Eye Institute
Professor of Clinical Ophthalmology
University of Cincinnati
Cincinnati, Ohio

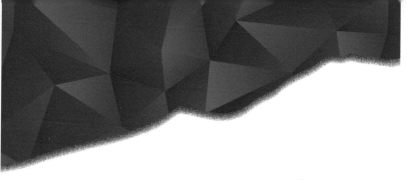

# Introduction

Microscopic surgery is unique in that you perform surgery without ever seeing your fingers. Most text-books on surgery focus on what is happening in the eye. In order to perform these objectives, it is important to know what your hands and fingers should be doing to facilitate this. That is the focus of this text.

The key to success in performing cataract surgery, cornea transplantation, and other anterior segment surgeries starts with the basics: how you hold your hands and how you hold the instruments in your hands. Once you put yourself in the most controlled position, the complication rates will diminish and it will be much easier for you to complete your steps in surgery.

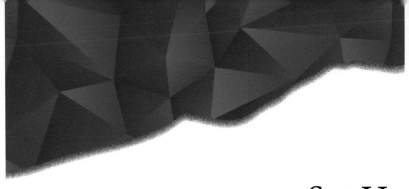

# Set Up

How you position yourself at the start of the case is very important. Our practice is to have our bodies at right angles: the tibia to femur, femur to spine, and humerus hanging freely (basically perpendicular) to the forearm. You should be comfortable in this position on the foot pedals and looking through the microscope.

Focus the microscope under the maximum magnification. The reason for this is to eliminate as much accommodation as you may have, which will affect the vision of your assistant and the video screen. Once set, you may adjust the magnification to what you desire. The video camera should remain in focus, meaning you have corrected for accommodation. Also make sure the oculars are adjusted to "Plano" and not to a minus or plus correction.

You will need to run the foot pedals with your feet. Our recommendation is that you put the phacoemulsification foot pedal under your right foot. Since we drive automobiles with our right foot on the accelerator, it is already adjusted to some of the skills your foot will be required to do, particularly with sophisticated surgical systems. This will give you a head start on these skills, and your left foot will need to learn how to work the microscope.

# Hand Position

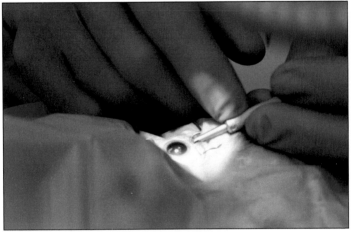

*Note the position of the finger on the head.*

The principle to use to achieve control and stability is by using your fifth metacarpal. This area of the hand is placed on the patient's head. Sometimes this is slanted more toward the first phalange depending on the facial structure and what you are trying to accomplish.

Establish this contact and your proprioception is anchored. This will allow you to use the instruments in a much more controlled fashion. If the patient's head should move, your hands are there on the head, allowing you to keep the instruments in the eye in the same relationship to the endothelium, lens, and vitreous. If there is a large movement, you are able to remove the instrument, minimizing the damage.

Movement of the head and eye complicate our attempts to do surgery, and we will address that further at the end of this manual.

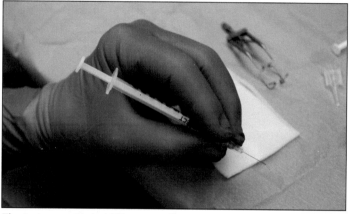

*The instrument is held like a pencil.*

The principle of holding the instrument is to hold it like a pencil in your thumb, index, and middle fingers. Once you have the instrument in that position, you can then practice to become more facile in how you hold it. For example, for different tasks, you may orient the instrument in a different way in those 3 digits.

Let's start with cataract surgery. The phacoemulsification handpiece is best held as a pencil. We recommend looping the cord in the crook of your elbow. If the cord moves, this can pull on the tip when it is inside the eye. You want to make sure you have eliminated this source of error by controlling it before you start.

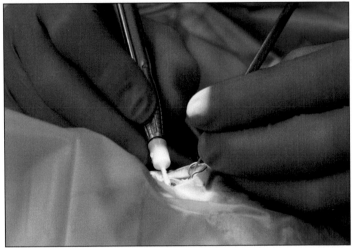

*Hand position for second instrument and phaco tip.*

For the purpose of this discussion, we will speak in terms of the right-handed surgeon. It would be reversed for the left-handed surgeon.

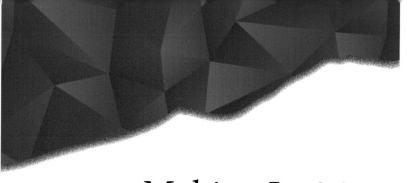

# Making Incisions

On setting up to the eye, your right and left hand will naturally come to certain locations on the eye. For the beginner, it is here that you want to make your incisions. The stab incision, or side port, is made first, with the knife held like a pencil. If it is made in the natural position, it will be very easy for you to find that incision without looking when it comes time to use a second instrument in the eye.

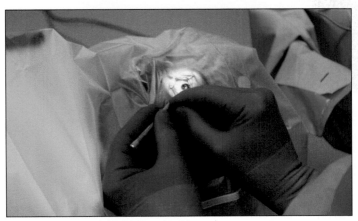

*Hand position for side port incision.*

Similarly, if you make your primary incision where the right hand comes to the eye, this will eliminate a source of torque and deformity of the wound. The deformity of the wound during surgery is the major cause of complications and the anterior chamber shallows, which makes capsulorrhexis, phacoemulsification, irrigation and aspiration, capsule polishing, and intraocular lens (IOL) insertion much more difficult.

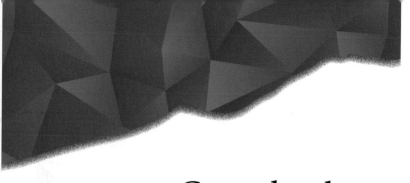

# Capsulorrhexis

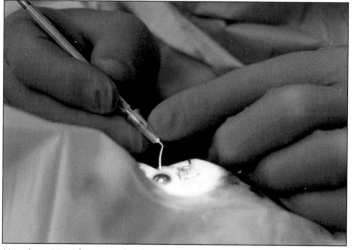

*Hand position for capsulorrhexis insertion of cystitome.*

The key to optimum control is to anchor the right hand (dominant hand) as described previously to hold the instrument. The left hand (nondominant hand) is also anchored.

The index finger of the left hand is used as fulcrum. The tip of the index finger is placed on the hub of the needle. The pivoting is then much more controlled. You are using your index finger to guide your movements, and this avoids deformity of the wound as you are able to keep the entry point stable while performing the surgery.

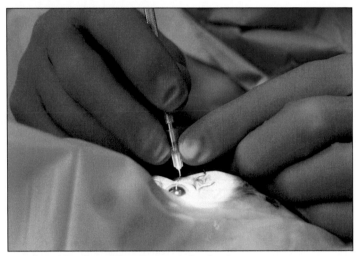

*Hand position for performing capsulorrhexis.*

# Injection of Fluids

It is very important that you hold the hub of the needle or cannula when you inject fluids into the eye. This is essential whether it is on a Luer lock syringe or not. The most important reason for doing this is so the needle does not fly into the eye under the pressure you have just put on the syringe. We have had the cannula suddenly release from Luer lock syringes. Since we had a hold on the hub of the cannula with the thumb and forefinger, the cannula did not release into the eye under pressure, saving a lot of distress for both surgeon and patient.

The other reason to hold the cannula in this way is that it allows you to rotate the cannula in the eye with the thumb and forefinger while injecting fluid. This gives you exceedingly good control while performing delicate tasks.

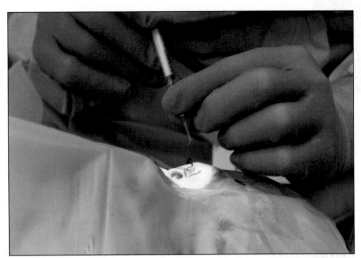

*Preparing to inject fluid to hydrodissect. Note how the hub of the cannula is secured.*

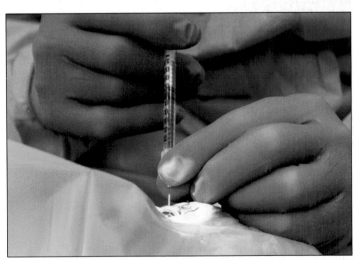

*Maneuvering the syringe using the hub of the cannula. Note the left hand position anchored to the head. The index finger and thumb are able to rotate the cannula.*

# Two-Handed Technique of Phacoemulsification

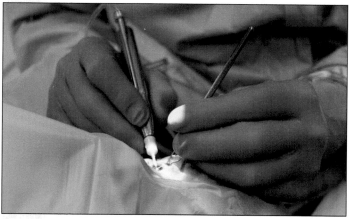

*The phaco tip is held as a pencil and the second instrument is held further down on the fourth finger to allow maneuvers inside the eye. The hands are anchored.*

This photo shows the hand position for a 2-handed technique of phacoemulsification. The phaco tip is held like a pencil in the right hand and the second instrument in the left is not. The hands are anchored to the head with the fourth and fifth metacarpals.

The instrument in the left hand is held differently by the fingers in order to accomplish a task without moving the hands. This is an important principle to grasp because if the left hand was to be off the head in this position, the instrument would not be well-controlled. The phaco tip is held like a pencil as these movements will basically be back and forth. The second instrument in the left hand will primarily be doing rotary movements, holding the instrument differently; resting in on the fourth finger allows this to occur much easier. By simply holding it differently with the fingers, stability and control are greatly improved.

# Irrigation and Aspiration

This is performed in the same manner as the capsulorrhexis. The tip of the index finger is used as the fulcrum, taking pressure off the wound, which could cause shallowing.

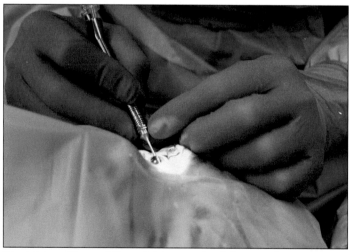

*The left hand is providing a fulcrum to the right to perform irrigation and aspiration.*

When performing irrigation and aspiration, the tip will be moving in 3 dimensions, including in a circular pattern. The index finger of the left hand is acting as a fulcrum on that side while the third finger of the right is performing the same function on the right.

The right hand will move from right to left and up and down while removing the cortex, and the previously mentioned fingers will help to stabilize the position of the tip in the eye. At a minimum, the fifth finger of the right hand (meaning the strongest position of the right hand is as shown, the weakest is just the right index finger in contact) will remain in contact with the head throughout this part of the procedure.

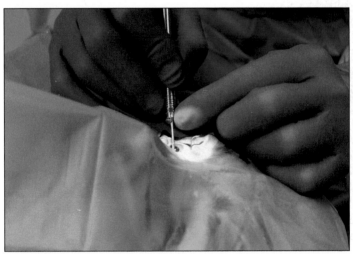

*Using the left index finger to stabilize the handpiece, the right hand has lifted significantly, anchored by the fifth finger. This is how you would aspirate viscoelastic under the IOL.*

# Placement of Viscoelastic

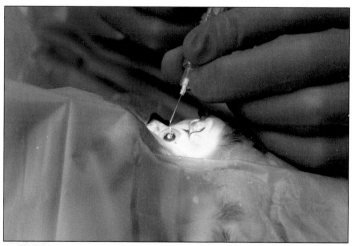

*By anchoring to the head and controlling the hub of the cannula, the surgeon has complete control in injecting viscoelastic.*

In the injection of viscoelastic, the left fingers control the hub of the cannula and the syringe while the dominant right hand injects. Notice how the left hand is firmly anchored to the head of the patient.

# Insertion of Intraocular Lens

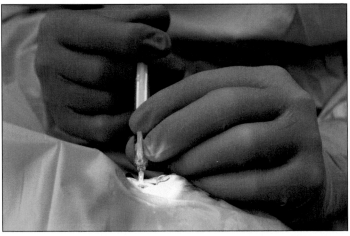

*The left hand stabilizes and positions the IOL injector while the right injects.*

The hand position here is similar to the injection of viscoelastic. Depending on the type of lens being inserted, a pushing or twisting action will be required of the right hand; this can involve significant force at times. Having the left hand firmly anchored again helps to stabilize.

# Retrobulbar Injection

The technique of retrobulbar injection is relatively simple but requires an understanding of what you are trying to achieve. For performing cornea transplants, for example, it is critical that there is only 3 cc of anesthetic in the muscle cone. If there is more than that (in general, not always), this can cause increased pressure on the globe, which becomes problematic once the cornea is off and the globe is completely open.

The visualization that you want is that of an ice cream cone. There is a scoop of ice cream—the globe—sitting on top of the muscle cone.

The principle is to push the scoop of ice cream up and out of the way and slide the needle into the cone. Remember, the scoop of ice cream will be of a different size in each patient. For this reason, use your index finger to locate the equator of the globe as you push it up.

The index finger identifies the orbital rim. So, the index finger is pushing the globe upward, which identifies the equator of the globe and, at the same time, has also identified the orbital rim. The needle is then inserted through the skin, past the equator, and on a line to the apex of the cone. This is a straight insertion; there is no changing of direction as you go. This is also not a fast motion; you slowly advance until you are past the equator. There is often a small resistance as you pass through the septum along the equator of the globe as you go through the cone. With the globe on the tip of the index finger, you know that the needle is not penetrating the globe.

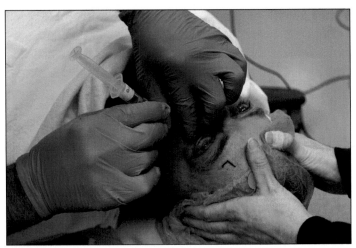

*The syringe is held in the right hand in a way similar to holding a dart. The globe is being pushed up, creating a space between the orbital rim and the globe.*

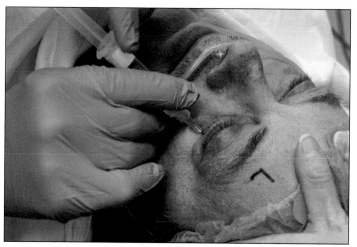

*The right hand is maintaining the position of the needle by being anchored to the patient's face. The left hand injects the anesthetic.*

The insertion of the needle has been in a straight line. Once in position, the left hand is used to inject the anesthetic while the right hand continues to hold the syringe while being anchored, providing stability.

There are some eyes in which the globe is very large and you cannot find the equator of the globe with your fingertip. It is these eyes that you can either place a peribulbar injection (ie, you are placing the anesthetic outside the muscle cone) or use a different approach in which you inject through the conjunctiva.

We have personally seen one case referred to us in which a retrobulbar injection was given that resulted in a choroidal hemorrhage, which became expulsive as the old cornea transplant wound gave way. Since this was an only eye, we replaced the contents and resutured the wound.

The patient, after retina consultation and no light perception vision, agreed to enucleation. In performing the enucleation, the globe completely filled the orbital cavity and was extremely difficult to remove.

In these large eyes in which you do not feel comfortable placing the needle behind the globe, the following technique is my preference. This was popularized by Greenbaum in 1999 with a special cannula that is no longer available. In its place, we use the 19-gauge cannula from the irrigation bottle. Using the operating microscope, the conjunctiva and tenons are opened in the fornix; this is done with Vannas scissors. A small dissection is performed until the space between the globe and tenons is visible. The cannula, now on a 3-cc syringe, is placed into this space and directed around the globe downward, and the anesthetic is injected. The conjunctiva will billow, and this can be massaged to push it more retrobulbar. It usually takes about 5 minutes to have a full effect.

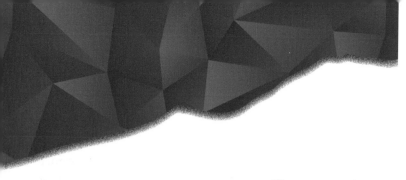

# Suturing

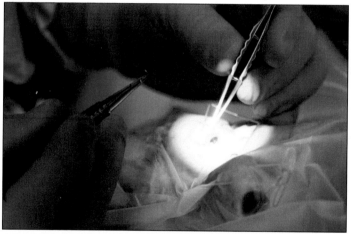

*A forward suture pass has been made; the fingers in the right hand have rotated forward around the thumb.*

It is important that the arc-shaped needle be grasped at about two-thirds of its length. This is the optimum location to place the suture in surgery. Too close to the suture material makes for a difficult pass and often a bent needle. Too close to the tip can result in an incomplete pass.

If it is not handed to you correctly, regrasp the needle. The best technique for this is as follows: hold the suture material well above the needle and let the needle rest on the corneal surface. Using the left hand, pirouette the needle so that it is perpendicular to the tip of the needle driver in the right hand. In this manner, you can grasp the needle exactly where you want with one attempt. Each time you touch the needle with the needle driver, magnetism occurs, which will cause the needle to move as you attempt to grasp it, similar to a compass needle being brought close to a magnet. This technique helps eliminate this, and you want to start with the needle properly loaded to maximize your success.

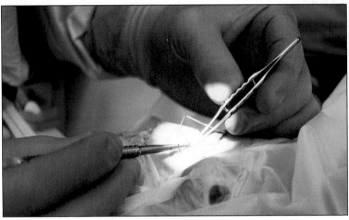

*A backhanded suture pass. The left hand has moved forward to grasp the tissue; the fingers of the right hand will rotate backward in relation to the thumb.*

A backhanded suture is being placed. The left hand has moved forward on the head to optimize its stability while maintaining its stability.

Notice how the angle of the Colibri forceps (Storz Ophthalmics) is changed by the position of the third finger and thumb. The third finger has pulled back toward the surgeon to achieve the angle to grasp the tissue without moving the hand.

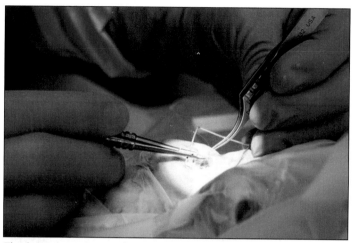

*The host tissue is now being grasped, and the fingers are rotating backward around the thumb to complete the pass.*

This shows that the angle of the forceps has changed dramatically without moving the hand. The third, fourth, and fifth fingers have not changed position, while the thumb and index have to achieve this angle.

Small-toothed forceps (our preference is a Colibri forceps) are used to evert the corneal wound edge. The needle tip is then generally placed at the fold just created by the forceps pulling back on the corneal tissue and pushed through to at least two-thirds depth (think of it as two-thirds cornea thickness).

The forceps then release the cornea side and grasp the host side. The needle has not been released at this point, and the appropriate depth at about roughly two-thirds is determined. The needle is initially slightly pushed into the tissue, but this is only microns. The second half of the pass is much different technically. It is not a push at all; it is a rotation. The needle is rotated following its natural arc in the following manner. Using the thumb to rotate upward and the middle finger to rotate downward, the needle driver is rotated in the fingers, thereby rotating the needle.

The needle driver is released at this point and the hub of the needle can be regrasped and rotated further if necessary. Ideally, you would like to reload the needle driver as the needle is held by the tissue. If you grab the tip of the needle, you will dull it, so you should avoid doing that.

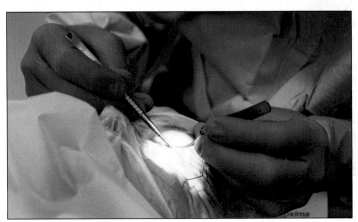

*This view has a broader perspective. The left hand appears to be off the head, but the third finger can be seen anchored. The fourth and fifth fingers are also touching the head.*

This is the hand position for a forward suture. Notice the left hand has moved its anchoring position completely and is much closer to the surgeon. This is the most common type of suture placed. Of importance here is how the needle driver is held by the right hand. You can see that the needle pass on the second half of the suture placement (in a cornea transplant, this would be into the host) can be easily accomplished by rotating the needle along its arc. The thumb and third finger of the right hand can rotate the needle driver for this portion of the pass while the index finger helps stabilize. The fourth and fifth finger and metacarpals provide an anchor to the head for much greater control.

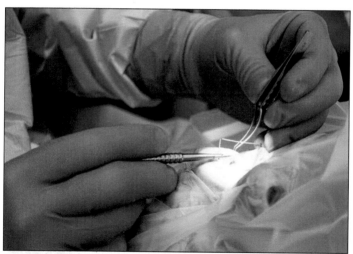

*A forward suture being placed. The first part of the suture pass is a push; the second will be rotation.*

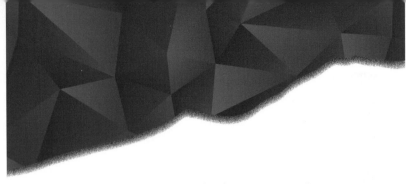

# Tying Sutures

For the right-handed surgeon, the biggest key to success in tying sutures is to have the suture coming up toward the microscope with the forceps held in the left hand. A Kelman-McPherson forceps is often used. This type of tying forceps has a long platform at an angle to the handle. This is not our preference; we prefer 2 straight-tying forceps.

The reason for this is that the straight instrument can be used to pick up the suture exactly as described, with the suture coming up toward the microscope. If you use a Kelman-McPherson forceps, it is often necessary to pick up the suture with the instrument in the right hand and then place it into the Kelman-McPherson. This is an extra step.

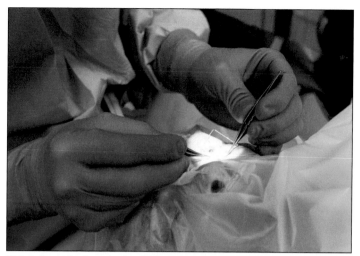

*This is how the hands should be positioned.*

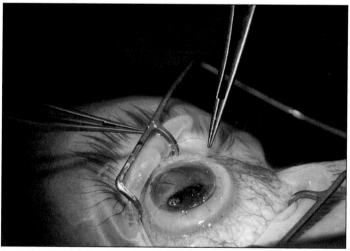

*In a close-up of the above image, the suture can be seen coming up and out of the tying forceps in the left hand.*

Once you have the suture coming up and out of the instrument in the left hand, you can then place 3 throws over the tying forceps in the right hand. Then you are right over the piece of suture that you want to pick up with the right hand. A little backward movement of the instrument in the left hand keeps the loops in place without tightening the loops so you cannot open the instrument in the right hand. Once the loose end of the suture is grasped in the right hand, the right instrument is brought toward the surgeon and the left instrument away, laying down the 3 throws, which can be snugged to the appropriate tension. The right instrument is then released, one throw placed, and the loose end regrasped. The instruments then move in the opposite direction. The tension on this second throw is to pull the previous throws into a ball. The first throw should have been linear. A final third throw is placed in a similar manner as the previous two. The suture can then be trimmed at the knot.

When tying the suture, the hands stay anchored as described. The fingers will move forward and backward over the knot.

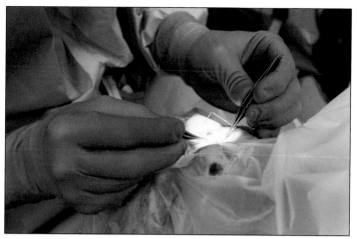

*The suture is being tied with a forward throw.*

The left hand has moved forward as the knot is tied and the tip of the tying forceps is below the eye. Note the position of the left hand.

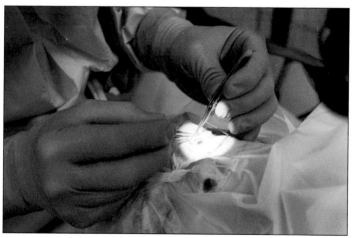

*The second throw has been made, and the suture is being picked up with the right tying forceps.*

The throw of the suture has now been made in the opposite direction; the tip of the tying forceps is now above the globe. The left index finger maintains its anchor to the globe, providing proprioception and stability. The hand has moved toward the surgeon to tie the knot.

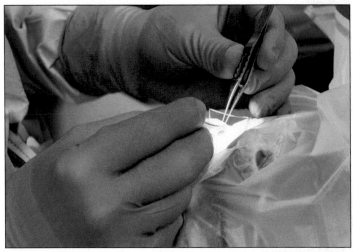

*Another throw is being tightened. The hands are starting to move in opposite directions.*

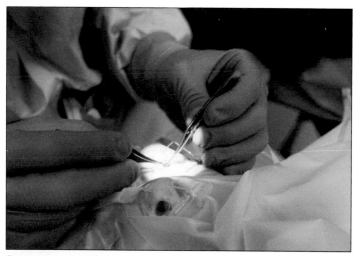

*Basic suturing technique.*

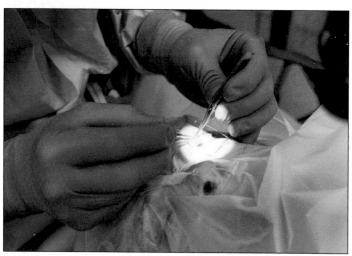

*Suturing, tying the knot. The left fifth finger is stabilizing the hand. Note that the left hand has moved significantly but the fifth finger has not.*

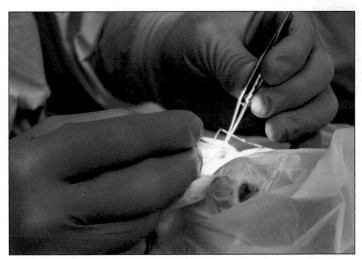

*This view shows the tip of the fifth finger providing stability as a suture in a difficult location is tied.*

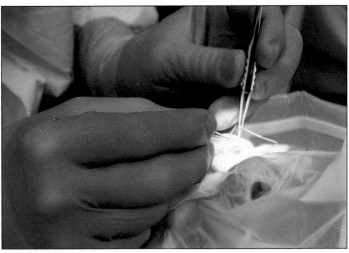

*Tying a suture in a different location, notice how the anchor finger has moved.*

# Advanced Techniques

As the surgery becomes more technical, the principle is that the hand position remains the same with regard to the fifth and fourth fingers and metacarpals, but the instrument is held in a completely different way.

We had previously mentioned that the instruments should be held as a pencil in each hand. There are certain situations in which you will want to alter how the instrument is held in your first 3 digits. For example, let's look at cornea transplantation. When you are excising a cornea button, the scissors will cut to the right and to the left depending on with which instrument you start. Keeping the fourth and fifth finger anchored in the same position but rotating your index and middle finger position around your thumb and chasing the angle of the instrument (ie, the base of the scissor away from your hand or the base of the scissor toward your hand like a pencil), you can make the incisions controlled and easy. This avoids having to switch hands, which is also an option and sometimes necessary.

This also gives you the facility to rise up off the head, using your ring and little finger as contact points to access difficult areas.

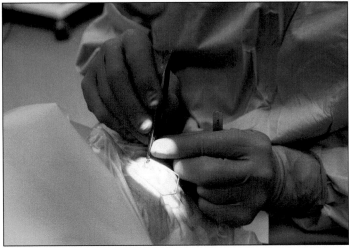

*Corneal scissors are used to cut the host tissue after trephination. The scissors are cutting down and to the left.*

The cornea button is being excised with scissors cutting to the right and down. The left index finger is providing stability as the right hand works the scissors.

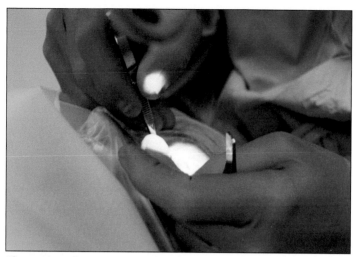

*These corneal scissors are cutting up and to the left. Notice the left hand anchored to the head and then providing a fulcrum for further control of the cut.*

The scissors are now cutting to the left and up. Notice the scissors held completely differently by the right hand. The left hand has moved to allow stability as well, and now it is more comfortable to use the third finger for this.

It sometimes takes some experimentation to find what works best for you, and it often necessitates placing the instrument in the right hand with the left.

# Movement of the Head and Eye

We have spent a great deal of time teaching you how to be stable and controlled through a wound during surgery. This presupposes that the wound itself is not moving in space. However, during cataract surgery in particular, the head and eye will move. If you are working on a left eye, for example, and the patient turns his or her head slightly away from you, this will create downward pressure on the wound and allow the chamber to shallow. The choices are either to follow the head by changing your wrist and hand angles accordingly or to stop and bring the head back into position.

The bells movement of rotating the eye up and out on closure will also tend to occur. This is usually much more obvious to detect, and similar compensations need to take place. The subtle movements of the head are not so easy to detect and can take place gradually.

If you are having difficulty maintaining chamber or controlling movements in the eye and your hand position is correct, consider removing your instruments and reassessing the head position. Sometimes, the patient will respond to a verbal command to put his or her chin down or turn his or her head slightly toward the surgeon, whatever the case may be.

As a starting surgeon, a retrobulbar block is helpful as you learn these techniques. In some patients, it may be very helpful, even for an experienced surgeon.

In conclusion, learning to do microsurgery is not easy and requires practice. It is our hope that showing you how to place your hands to give you the most stability and control will shorten your road to mastery.

Printed in the United States
by Baker & Taylor Publisher Services